An Easy Way
To Understand
Erectile Dysfunction
(Impotence)

Also By Brian B Jacques

His very popular Series of Mini-Health Books includes:

- An Easy Way To Understand Eczema and Psoriasis
- An Easy Way To Understand Stress and Depression
- An Easy Way To Understand Vitamins and Minerals
- An Easy Way To Understand Parasites, Worms, Candida, Constipation & Detoxing
- An Easy Way To Understand Crohn's Disease and IBD
- An Easy Way To Understand Body Building For Men And Women
- An Easy Way To Understand Alzheimer's Disease
- An Easy Way To Understand Herpes
- An Easy Way To Understand Parkinson's Disease
- An Easy Way To Understand Autism
- An Easy Way To Understand Fibromyalgia
- An Easy Way To Understand Your Body Systems
- An Easy Way To Understand Erectile Dysfunction
- An Easy Way To Understand Heart Disease, High Blood Pressure & Stroke
- An Easy Way To Understand Detoxing For Men & Women
- How To Lose Weight After 40
- How To Lose Weight And Maintain Your Ideal Weight Permanently
- Amino Acids & Enzymes—What Are They & Why Do You Need Them
- The Little A–Z Dictionary of Herbal Remedies
- The Magic Of Vitamins & Minerals
- Effective Methods To Stop Smoking
- Eat Wholefoods And Take Supplements—The Ultimate Lifestyle Guide
- Stress Busters Adult Coloring Book

All these books are available as Kindle Editions (available from the Kindle Store on Amazon.com, and other countries Amazon sites where the Kindle platform is supported.) Many of these books are also available for the Barnes and Noble "Nook". In addition, many of these titles are available as print editions from the Amazon website.

An Easy Way To Understand Erectile Dysfunction (Impotence)

Brian B Jacques

Wisdom For Life Media

"Education is the kindling of a flame, not the filling of a vessel." —Socrates

Contents

Acknowledgment

To the many people I have come into contact with throughout my life, whose belief in me has made everything possible and worthwhile.

1. Diagnosis

Do you get an unexpected ejaculation during intercourse? If you do, this can raise all kinds of fears in your mind—the uppermost being that you may have erectile dysfunction (ED), or to give it its more common name—impotence. Even though the act of intercourse may have been satisfactory, doubts linger in your mind.

Fluctuations in your hormones will occur naturally, and are nothing to be alarmed about. In addition, a failure to achieve regular nocturnal erections is also another reason to fear the worst.

So what is the best thing to do? A visit to your doctor or to a licensed sexual health clinic is required. This way, you will get a proper diagnosis of your condition, and if there is a problem, then how severe is it, and how to treat it?

Whilst the diagnosis is being undertaken, it is important that you are open and honest about what you feel is wrong. This way, you will be able to get an accurate diagnosis. It is important not to be shy and reserved in your discussion with your doctor. Remember, they have dealt with symptoms of erectile dysfunction many times before so there is nothing to be afraid of.

During your health assessment, your doctor will determine if emotional, psychological or physiological issues are involved, because if they are, then, medication for a possible erectile dysfunction problem is not going to help. For these issues you could be referred to a therapist or counselor, who will arrange various sessions with you, to help determine if there are any underlying concerns which could be affecting your sexual performance.

Your doctor will ask questions to get an overall picture of your sexual history. It can be an advantage to take your partner along as well, as her input can be really valuable in getting an overall picture of your sexual activity.

You will be asked questions about your overall health and any medications you are prescribed for existing medical conditions will be assessed. If you are overweight, suffer from diabetes and/or heart disease then your chances of having erectile dysfunction increase dramatically. You will be asked about your lifestyle, what type of work you do and if you are under stress or worry a lot.

Blood work will be undertaken—especially to determine your testosterone level. Also a urine test will be done as well as a serum test. Your prolactin levels will be measured, in addition to you lipid profile.

The results of these tests can help determine if you have erectile dysfunction. Aside from existing medical conditions, one of the main causes of erectile dysfunction is a low testosterone level—especially as you get older. If low testosterone is diagnosed in your case, then there are several ways to increase it. See the chapter on testosterone.

In addition to testosterone treatment you may also be prescribed Viagra, Levitra or Cialis to take just before sexual activity.

A Nocturnal Penile Tumescence (NPT) test may be suggested. Nocturnal erections happen in men of all ages and this denotes healthy sexual behavior. This is a very important test, and specially designed NPT labs conduct the sleep trial and do the evaluation on erection activity.

The important issue here is—if you think you have a problem with getting or maintaining an erection, then effective treatments are available for men of all ages. There is a caveat though. If you suffer from certain medical conditions—obesity, heart disease or diabetes— and take medications for those conditions, then this might make it more difficult to get or maintain an erection. And medications for erectile dysfunction may react adversely with medications you are taking for other health conditions. However, it is worthwhile discussing all these issues with your doctor.

2. Are You At Risk For Erectile Dysfunction

Please be aware that all men are at risk of developing erectile dysfunction, whatever your age. However, following a healthy lifestyle and having annual medical check-ups will lessen you risk of developing this condition. If you look after yourself, then there is no reason why you should not be able to get and maintain an erection well into your 70's and beyond. Unfortunately, age is a factor that increases your risk of developing erectile dysfunction.

The majority of men will observe a decline in their sexual drive as they get older. They will often find it more difficult to get an erection, and it will not last as long as it used to do. Additionally, as a person ages they are more at risk of developing medical conditions which can affect their erection capabilities. So, as mentioned above it is important to remain as healthy as you can, for as long as you can.

Men who fail to get an annual medical check-up increase their risk of developing erectile dysfunction. Such medical conditions as heart disease, hypertension (high blood pressure), low blood pressure, obesity, diabetes and high cholesterol are just a few of the medical conditions that can prevent you from achieving an adequate erection. Interestingly, men are less likely to get medical check-ups than women. But they do become increasingly important as you get older.

If a medical condition is diagnosed early enough, then there is a possibility that you may not have to take medication on a daily basis. Certain medications do interfere with your ability to get an erection. It could be a difficult choice between taking your medication for a medical condition, and being able to pursue an active sex life.

Where there is a genetic medical condition involved such as heart disease or diabetes, then this will automatically put you at an increased risk for erectile dysfunction. If you are aware of a genetic link, then it is wise to see you doctor on a regular basis so he or she can monitor your overall health.

You may not have heard of a health condition called metabolic syndrome, but it is implicated in erectile dysfunction. This condition is caused by excess fat in the belly region, high cholesterol and high blood pressure. If you have any of these conditions, then it is important to work with your doctor to minimize you risk of developing erectile dysfunction.

Are you involved in what can be classed as dangerous sports? Sports such as wrestling, and football should only be undertaken with a protective cup in place. Any injuries you sustain to the spine or genital area can interrupt the flow of blood to your penis—which is essential to obtain an erection.

Do you ride a bike? If so, then you could be at risk for erectile dysfunction due to pressure from the bike seat. If you ride long distances, do you get numbness in the genital area? If so, you need to change the bike seat for one that is more suitable for you.

Your lifestyle can play a key role in your sexual activity. If you drink excessive amounts of alcohol, eat a diet that is high in fat, get very little exercise or smoke, then you increase your risk for developing erectile dysfunction.

It is never too late to make changes in your lifestyle. Changing your diet to a healthier one is not all that difficult to do. But changing a "habit" such as smoking or drinking may need the help of a support group.

If you have done very little exercise before, then it is important to discuss this with your doctor before you start, to make sure that the exercise program you propose doing is right for you, especially is if you have a medical condition. All the suggestions in this chapter are worthwhile if you want to maintain a healthy sex life.

You have to do your part to make sure that you do not join the ever growing statistics of those who suffer from erectile dysfunction. By not abusing your body you will help to ensure that you stay healthy and enjoy more than just a good sex life with your partner.

There are a multitude of risk factors that can have a bearing on your sexual health. Many of these factors you can control yourself through your lifestyle choices—so always make sure that you listen to what your body is telling you.

3. Statistics

The latest estimates suggest that roughly 30 million men globally have erectile dysfunction. The estimates suggest that roughly half, 50 percent have had the condition professionally diagnosed. The sad part is that a large proportion of the other 50 percent often feel too embarrassed to discuss it with either a medical professional or their partner—in other words, they hide the condition.

Analyzing the statistics shows that 1 in 10, men have had to pick up the courage to deal with the problem. The common belief is that only older men suffer from erectile dysfunction. However, this is not the case. This condition can affect men of all ages. Interestingly, only 40 percent of men who have been professionally diagnosed are over the age of 40. The rest are much younger.

Certain medical conditions can cause men to suffer from this condition, the main ones being diabetes and heart disease. Statistics show that half (50 percent) of men with diabetes will ultimately suffer from erectile dysfunction. If you suffer from diabetes it is important to get it under control, to help reduce the risk of developing erectile dysfunction in the future.

Smoking can put you at significant risk of developing erectile dysfunction. Smoking just one pack each day will increase your risk of developing this condition by 50 percent. And smoke more than one pack each day and your risk factor triples. For older men, the risk significantly increases as each year goes by.

Men seem to be more ready to admit they have a problem when they complete online surveys, or with surveys where they can remain anonymous. In these anonymous surveys nearly 56 percent of men admitted that they have a problem gaining an erection, and keeping it. One short-coming of the surveys is that the level of severity cannot be determined. But the surveys show that these men need to see their doctor to discuss an effective treatment program for their condition.

When considering what treatments are available, the majority of men appeared to be very familiar with prescription drugs. Of some concern, a large majority—89 percent said that despite all the risks, side effects, allergy reactions and health warnings they would take a prescription medication if it would solve their erectile dysfunction problem. The reason that the majority of men gave for taking prescription medications was that their ability to perform sexually is a key part of being a man and of a satisfying life with their partner.

Over 600,000 men are seen each year by medical professionals due to problems with erectile dysfunction. This statistic can indicate that more men than ever before are suffering from this problem. One positive thing though is that with all the educational information available, more men than ever are seeking assistance and treatment for their condition. They are now more aware than ever that treatment options are available to them.

As more men begin to realize the importance of seeking help and professional care, the statistics hopefully will become more reliable, with the result that a better picture will emerge of how big a problem this condition really is in society as a whole.

It is important to understand that for 90 percent of men, there is an effective treatment available for them—all they need to do is seek medical attention, get all their questions answered, and have either the correct medication prescribed for them, or if the condition is emotional or psychologically based, then have a treatment plan devised by a licensed professional..

4. Emotional And Psychological Problems

For a significant number of men, erectile dysfunction is not associated with any health problem but is in fact the result of emotional or psychological problems that the individual is experiencing or has experienced in the past. It is important to understand that in order for a man to achieve an erection signals have to be sent to the nerves from the brain. Therefore, if the messages being sent are not what they should be, the end result will not be what is expected.

Stress is one of the major factors when it comes to erectile dysfunction. It can be difficult to concentrate on sexual activities when you have other things on your mind. In reality, it is very difficult to eliminate all stress from your life; however, you can certainly take steps to reduce it. You need to take a careful look into all aspects of your life. If stress continues to be a major issue due to work, relationships, finances or other concerns then you need to take steps to find solutions to your problems.

Some men feel that they are under too much pressure to perform sexually. They may have a great desire to be with someone, but they may suffer from low self-esteem. The consequence of this is that they have an excessive amount of anxiety concerning how they will perform in the eyes of the other person. Such expectations can lead to erectile dysfunction. And what makes matters worse is that some men have been belittled by partners from previous relationships, so their confidence is not high in their ability to perform and sexually satisfy the person they are with now.

Being over tired can also result in erectile dysfunction. This is often viewed as a physical problem, and while this might be true in some cases, it is not true in all. It is possible for a man to feel mentally exhausted. This most commonly happens when a serious situation has happened. For example emotional strain that comes after the loss of a loved one, a divorce or even the loss of a job. Additionally, depression can also result in erectile dysfunction.

If a man has been sexually abused as a child this can have life-long effects. Sometimes these events can be buried deep in the subconscious. On occasions when a man becomes of age and starts to become sexually active these buried emotions can trigger emotional responses which can make it difficult to maintain an erection. This type of experience is very difficult to overcome—but it can be done.

Some men are brought up in an environment that emphasizes it is improper to have sexual intercourse unless they are married. These ideals may be promoted by the family or as part of religious doctrine. Either way a psychological dilemma can be created in an individual which then has to be dealt with. Even if the person doesn't realize that internal conflicts are present it can in fact result in erectile dysfunction.

Arranging sessions with a therapist or counselor can help you identify various emotional and psychological problems that could be causing your erectile dysfunction. For these sessions to be successful it is very important to be open and honest. Patience is also needed as it can take some time to explore inner thoughts and feelings.

For some men having counseling sessions with their partner is very therapeutic. The answers to problems with the man's erectile dysfunction could be found within the relationship itself. As an example, some men find it very difficult to maintain an erection after their partner has cheated on them. In addition, there may be buried anger concerning other aspects of the relationship that have not yet been shared.

Understanding that emotional and psychological problems can be the cause of your erectile dysfunction is an important consideration. You could start by seeing your doctor to make sure there are no medical conditions that could be causing the problem. During the medical assessment, it can often be determined if it is emotional or psychological problems that need to be addressed.

Accepting the advice of your doctor can often start you on a positive path to get your sex life back on track.

5. Heart Disease And Erectile Dysfunction

We tend to think of heart disease as a medical condition that mainly affects people as they age—however, it is now a condition that affects younger people as well.

So why has heart disease remained the major killer in most Western societies? There are several reasons: the main one being the Western diet which has low fiber content and is high in saturated fat, sugar and sodium as well as various additives and artificial colors and flavorings.

Lifestyle is another factor. The fast paced lifestyle which everyone seems to live by these days does not help the body to rebuild itself, with the end result that circulatory problems which we usually associate with heart disease and stroke have freedom to destroy the body; and couple this with a stressful lifestyle due to work and family demands, and we have a recipe for disaster.

I often get asked what heart disease has to do with erectile dysfunction. In fact, it has a lot to do with it. Many people think that blocked arteries caused by arterial plaque are the main cause of a heart attack—and whilst this is partly true, there are other factors which can lead to heart disease.

But consider this, one of the causes of erectile dysfunction is arteries that feed blood to the penis which stimulates an erection, also get blocked with plaque, which in turn leads to a restricted blood flow, which has an impact on a male being able to get or sustain an erection.

Hypertension (high blood pressure) is often linked to heart disease. This has the effect of decreasing the elasticity of the arteries that not only supply blood to the heart but to every other part of the body—including the penis. As a consequence, high blood pressure leads to inadequate pressure in the penile tract which can cause difficulties in maintaining an erection for a sustained period of time.

Therefore as you can see from the above heart disease and erectile dysfunction are linked. If you suffer from heart disease, then it is highly probable that you suffer from erectile dysfunction as well;

conversely, if you suffer from erectile dysfunction, then you should see your doctor to get yourself checked out to see if there is any underlying heart disease condition. Always remember that heart disease can kill you, but erectile dysfunction cannot.

If a person is taking medication for heart disease, then careful consideration has to be taken by your doctor before any medications for erectile dysfunction can be prescribed. Some heart disease medications when combined with those for erectile dysfunction can reduce blood pressure to a dangerously low level. If this is the case, then, your doctor would caution against taking medications for erectile dysfunction—which is not what you would probably want to hear. However, there are other remedies that can be considered which I have explained elsewhere in this book.

I also mentioned stress earlier in this chapter. Stress can be implicated in erectile dysfunction; therefore any medications which have been prescribed for this condition can have a beneficial effect on erectile dysfunction as well.

There is a gland in the brain known as the hypothalamus, which gets all excited by stress and sends out panic messages to all the other glands in the body. It sends out alarms to the pituitary gland, which in turn sends further messages to the nervous systems and the adrenal glands. These churn out stress hormones which not only put a severe strain on the body but also on your mind as well.

Over time it just gets worse and worse as more and more of what are basically killer substances move around the body. These can lead to chronic conditions not only heart-related but different cancers, a reduced immune system which is not as effective in combating disease, allergies—and of course stress itself. And all of this can affect your ability to gain an adequate erection and keep your penis hard for the required amount of time.

Therefore, trying to relax and reduce your stress levels can be very beneficial, as can getting adequate exercise to reduce your stress levels, and also consider making changes to your diet.

To sum up: There is a direct correlation between heart disease, stress, hypertension (high blood pressure) and erectile dysfunction. Discussing these issues with your doctor cannot only increase your lifespan, but it can also enhance your erection abilities as well.

6. Testosterone Therapy

Testosterone is the male sex hormone, which is responsible for sexual characteristics and activity. As you get older, testosterone levels tend to decline. And because of this decline, erectile dysfunction can become a problem. However, this condition is treatable and in this chapter we will discuss testosterone therapy.

Testosterone deficiency can be characterized as low sexual drive and the loss of interest in sexual activity. Other indications of a low testosterone level include: increased body fat, decreased muscle mass, reduced body hair mass, and in some cases brittle bones. Low testosterone levels can be treated with some of the therapies discussed below.

• **Intramuscular injections:** this involves injecting the testosterone directly into muscle tissue. This has the effect of allows the medication to be absorbed quickly into the blood stream. The medication can be injected into the shoulder, upper arm, thigh or buttocks. Your doctor will explain to you how to do the injections. If you feel that you cannot do this yourself, then a nurse in your doctor's office will do it for you, but you will need to visit every one to four weeks. Do not inject testosterone into a vein.

• **Testosterone patch:** this is one method that may be suggested by your doctor. The patch is placed as directed and stimulates the production of testosterone and it can be effective in some individuals.

• **Testosterone gel:** this is probably the easiest and most effective ways of treating testosterone deficiency. It is usually applied on top of the shoulders or for more rapid absorption—under the armpits.

Your doctor will discuss with you whether to try the patch or the gel first. If these aren't successful, then the intramuscular injections will be suggested.

If you are prescribed testosterone treatment, then it is important to get a Prostate-Specific Antigen (PSA) blood test done every three months to detect any early signs of prostate cancer. You do have a slightly increased risk of prostate cancer if you use testosterone replacement medications. Your doctor will do the test for you and assess the result. If your PSA is normal then the treatment can be continued indefinitely.

Brian B Jacques

7. Levitra

The erectile dysfunction medication Levitra doesn't seem to get as much attention in the media as does Cialis or Viagra. This lack of attention may lead many men to believe that it is not a very effective treatment. However, if you do some research into Levitra, you will find that many men get a very positive benefit from taking it.

If you decide to give it a try, your doctor will probably start you on a low dose of 2.5mg. If this dose proves ineffective then it can be increased to a maximum of 20mg. A man should not take more than one dose in a 24 hour period. This medication has been approved by the Food and Drug Administration (FDA) for use in cases of erectile dysfunction.

Many men have been able to get and maintain a satisfactory erection using Levitra, even if they have been unsuccessful using other similar types of medication. It is important to understand that whist many erectile dysfunction medication are similar they are all different in some way. So, while one may not work, Levitra might. It is therefore worthwhile giving it a try if you haven't done so already.

The normal time scale for a man to achieve an erection after taking Levitra is 30 minutes. Many men report an added benefit of getting an erection that lasts longer and is firmer than it used to be. These additional benefits are not always experienced with other types of erectile dysfunction medications. Therefore these additional positive benefits are worth considering, and may be you would want to try Levitra to see if you can experience these additional benefits too.

Like most medications, there are some side effects including headaches, nausea and muscle pain. These side effects should subside in time. If you experience blurred vision or loss of hearing then you should discontinue using Levitra and consult your doctor.

Men that take nitrates for chest pains and heart disease should not take Levitra. This is because when these two types of medication are combined it can cause a drop in blood pressure to unsafe levels which could trigger a heart attack or stroke. Additionally, men who take alpha blockers for their prostate should not take Levitra.

Your doctor will have to do a medical evaluation of any existing medical conditions such as heart disease, diabetes, hypertension (high blood pressure) and high cholesterol.

Provided that any existing medical conditions are kept under control, then your doctor may give you the go-ahead to try Levitra, but a regular evaluation will be required to make sure there could be no negative outcomes. In some cases, medications taken for the medical conditions mentioned above can be taken along with Levitra. It is important to understand that each case has to be assessed on its individual merits.

Levitra is a very effective medication for men suffering from erectile dysfunction, but it is not for everyone! The first step is to talk to your doctor to see if this particular medication will be of benefit to you. Erectile dysfunction is treatable, so there is no need to go on suffering and not enjoying your sex life. Why not consider Levitra, if other types of similar medications have failed?

8. Viagra (Sildenafil)

Viagra—or to give it its generic name Sildenafil has been the top-selling product and the most popular for erectile dysfunction since it was first introduced in 1998. Approximately 80% of men who take it find that it is an effective treatment. Viagra is heavily advertised on TV and in magazines and it achieves billions of dollars each year in sales.

Erectile dysfunction used to be a subject that was not talked about because of fear or embarrassment. Now many men are prepared to provide their own testimonials of the benefits they have achieved from this product. You can find many of their statements on the Internet where men are prepared to help others that are in the same situation that they once were. And promoting Viagra is one way that they can achieve this.

If your doctor feels that Viagra could help you, then he or she will start you on the lowest dose which is 20 mg. This is one way your doctor can monitor how your body responds to the medication. The dose can be increased until you are achieving the desired results from it. The maximum dose is 100 mg and should this high dosage not achieve satisfactory results for you, then possibly, Viagra is not a suitable medication for you.

However, Viagra is a very effective treatment, and the majority of men will find that they can achieve a full erection within 30 minutes of taking it. You only take Viagra when you're ready for sexual activity to take place. As there is no cure for erectile dysfunction if it cannot be associated with a medical condition, then taking Viagra can help a man have a very satisfying sex life.

Viagra could prove unsuitable for someone with certain medical conditions including heart disease, high or low blood pressure, or diabetes. It is therefore important to discuss your medical condition with your doctor if you are considering taking this medication.

Never consider buying Viagra on the Internet or trying pills that have been prescribed for someone else. Your doctor will need to give you a full medical assessment before prescribing Viagra. It is therefore important that you feel confident to discuss your erectile dysfunction condition at this time.

In addition your doctor will want to rule out any physical and / or psychological problems that may be responsible for your erectile dysfunction. If either of these conditions is determined to be the root cause of the problem, then Viagra is not going to help, but other treatment options could.

There are various side effects associated with taking Viagra; however, most of these will subside as the body adjusts to the medication. In addition, your healthcare provider may be able to advise you about some of the ways of helping prevent or reduce some of these side effects. So here are the most common side effects: aches and pains in the muscles, nose bleeds, breathing difficulties, headache, skin redness, sneezing, and stomach discomfort after meals, stuffy or runny nose, difficulty sleeping and finally unnaturally warm skin.

There are other types of erectile dysfunction medications or treatment options available, some of these I have described elsewhere in this book, but Viagra remains the best-known brand and treatment for this condition. In addition, it has also provided a pathway for other erectile dysfunction medications to be developed.

9. The Benefits Of Cialis (Tadalafil)

Cialis—or to give it its generic name Tadalafil—is one of the most popular prescription medications for men suffering from erectile dysfunction. It is getting very positive reviews from men that use it; in fact, there is a strong possibility that it could outsell the market leader Viagra before too long. It is important not to think of all erectile dysfunction medications as being the same. They are all different in some way, and Cialis has many benefits that Viagra doesn't have, and this could be possibly why it receives so much attention.

Cialis is available in two different forms. So you can discuss with your doctor which one will be the best for you to take. If you plan on engaging in sexual activity a couple of times a week, then your doctor will recommend taking a pill before the event. This type of pill will allow you to engage in sexual activity for a period of 36 hours after taking it. This provides quite a window of opportunity to engage in a more spontaneous act than is available by taking other types of erectile dysfunction medication.

If you like to indulge in sexual activity on a more frequent basis then a daily pill is what you need. It is available in a low dose of either 2.5 mg or 5 mg. It is best to take it at the same time each day to achieve maximum benefits. This is a very good way for you to be able to achieve a normal sex life again. All it takes is to swallowing a pill at the same time each day.

The majority of men discover that Cialis has fewer side effects than other types of erectile dysfunction medications. Side effects can always be a concern with any type of medication, especially if it interferes with your daily activities. Taking a low dose Cialis will mean that the majority of side effects will not be a problem.

It is important to bear in mind that Cialis won't automatically give you an erection. You still need to be mentally or physically stimulated in order for it to occur. This will be a relief for many men as they don't want to walk around with a permanent erection. You will find that because of the stimulation needed there will be no embarrassing moments.

Existing medical conditions can always be a concern when considering which type of erectile dysfunction medication to take.

With Cialis as long as your doctor determines that you are healthy enough for sexual activity then you should be able to take this medication. If you have high blood pressure or diabetes then provided it is under control, your doctor may approve your use of this medication.

Unfortunately insurance companies usually don't pay for erectile dysfunction medications. So this can be an issue when trying to fit this type of medication into your budget. One piece of good news, Cialis is less expensive than Levitra or Viagra. But because it is cheaper doesn't mean it won't work. Many men will bear testimony to the effectiveness of Cialis by having a healthy normal sex life again.

So why is Cialis less-expensive? One reason is a lot of the initial research was already done when this medication was approved by the FDA. As a consequence, improvements could be made to a product that was already available. Another reason is that vast amounts of money are not spent on advertising. This could be one reason why the product is less well known, but it does have is devoted band of followers.

Cialis can provide some great benefits for anyone who suffers from erectile dysfunction. So why not talk to your doctor to discover if Cialis could be a beneficial treatment for you. The majority of men discover that Cialis is very effective and gives a great boost to their sex life. They get all the benefits with very little inconvenience to themselves.

10. Why Are Certain Drugs Effective

After other causes have been ruled out for a man's erectile dysfunction problem, then medications are the other pathway to go. As discussed in other chapters, the three most popular ones are Cialis, Levitra and Viagra. Whilst each of these is specific for treating erectile dysfunction, they each have significant differences. And it might be that a trial and error approach may be required in order to ultimately be prescribed the right one for you, so that you will be able to get an active sex life again.

These classes of drugs are known as PDE inhibitors. How they work is that when a man takes one of them, his body is able to use nitric oxide more effectively to relax muscles in the penis. The effect of this is that blood is able to flow more rapidly into the penile area for an erection to occur. At the same time, enzymes—which make the penis go limp—are blocked. The effect of this is that many men claim that their erections last longer, and that their penis is harder than it ever was. A man can get an erection within 30 minutes of taking it.

A major benefit is that a man has to be mentally and / or physically stimulated in order for the medication to work. There is no need to worry that they will have to walk around all day with an erection just because they are taking medication for their erectile dysfunction problem. Another benefit is that there is usually a 36 hour time frame when sexual activity can take place—giving you plenty of time to set the scene for a great sexual adventure with your partner.

Very strict guidelines have been set by the FDA for erectile dysfunction medications. Your doctor has to give you a complete medical examination to make sure no other conditions are causing the problem. This way, it can be determined if the patient is going to get a benefit from taking the medication or not. There are certain medical conditions where sexual activity would be unsuitable, in which case these types of medication would not be prescribed.

There is a lot of research available about the effectiveness of these types of medications. The success rate is high with men from all backgrounds. Even though there can be some initial side effects, most men are prepared to put up with the temporary inconvenience in order to have a good sex life again.

Further research and development is being undertaken to develop new drugs for this condition. This is positive news in that men who are prescribed these types of drugs will always receive the benefits of the latest developments.

The market for erectile dysfunction medicine is huge, and is far too significant for pharmaceutical manufacturers to ignore it.

11. Why Are Erectile Dysfunction Medications So Expensive

Let me start my giving you an example. A man has been struggling with erectile dysfunction for some time, so he finally gets up enough courage to go and see his doctor. After his doctor has given him the appropriate medical tests, he is told that his condition is not emotional or psychologically based, and yes, you can be helped; there is a prescription medication that could work for me.

So image this man's relief and delight when he has been told this. Now he is told the price of the medication—and all that motivation and excitement gets shot out of the sky. He asks the doctor to repeat the price, and he realizes that this could be way out of reach for him, as his monthly budget is rather tight as it is. So he has several choices to make: find the money somehow, purchase untried medications on the black market, or forget it altogether and put up with the condition.

And there is another problem. It is very unlikely that your health insurance plan will cover the cost of this type of medication. If your plan does cover it, then there could be a hefty deductive and / or co-pay associated with them. However, it is always worth checking with your insurance company. In fact insurance companies are getting more requests for this type of medication, and some of them may consider including it in their plans.

It is estimated that there are 160 million men out there with an erectile dysfunction problem. But only a small percentage will go and see their doctor to see what treatments are available. Many will prefer to go on the internet and purchase cheap, untested medications, either because of the high cost of prescription medications and / or to avoid the embarrassment of having to discuss it with their doctor. Remember, unlicensed medications could put your health at risk, especially if you have medical conditions that you are already taking prescription drugs for.

It is important to understand that economic forces are at work with erectile dysfunction medications—just like they are with other medications as well. Drug companies are in business to make a profit. There is a heavy financial investment in any type of medication through years of research and development before they are approved for patient use. And the drug companies have to recoup that investment. In addition, they will also continue to do additional research to enhance the benefits of their products—and this is especially true of erectile dysfunction medications.

Besides the research and development investment, there is also advertising costs to factor in. TV commercials are expensive, as are color ads in magazines and infomercials. There is also the cost of promoting their products within the medical community, and if they hire a celebrity to endorse their products, then that can cost a huge sum of money. And finally, the drug company will add on a percentage for their profit. Bear in mind that all these costs have to be factored into the price of the product that is ultimately paid by the patient.

Additionally, let us not forget the "perceived value" of an erectile dysfunction medication. As an example Cialis is one of the least expensive erectile dysfunction medications. You would imagine that because of the lower price many men would want to try it. But no! The perception is because it is cheaper, then it is inferior in some way—when in reality many men get tremendous benefits from taking it.

And because Viagra and Levitra are more expensive, then these two medications must be better. It is a lot to do with the "psychology of selling", and drug companies are well aware that if they drop the price of their more expensive medications, then the "perceived value" quantile is diminished, and they could lose patients.

With ever growing demand for erectile dysfunction products, and the ongoing research for more products for this condition, hopefully, the costs will decrease. Competition from new products coming into the market could force down prices. Currently there are only a few erectile dysfunction medications approved by the Food and Drug Administration (FDA). While this situation continues, prices will remain high and in some ways, quite cynically, drug manufacturers know that men will pay the high price to continue to enjoy a good sex life.

12. Treatment Devices

If testosterone therapy and erectile dysfunction medications do not work, or you have a medical condition that precludes you from taking medications for your condition, then your doctor may suggest one of two different devices which are outlined below.

Vacuum Constriction Device (VCD)

This device consists of an external pump with a band on it that can be used to obtain and maintain an erection.

The device consists of an acrylic cylinder with a pump that is attached to the end of the penis. A constriction ring or band is placed on the cylinder at the other end which is applied to the body. The cylinder and pump are used to suck air out and thus create a vacuum. The vacuum created draws extra blood into the penis making it erect. You then use the band or constriction ring to keep the erection and prevent blood from escaping back into the body.

Bear in mind that the pump has no lasting effect on the size of the penis. Once the band is removed, the penis will deflate.

What are the risks?

These include bruises, blisters, ruptured blood vessels and possibly thickened and discolored skin. The band should not be left in place for longer than 20 to 30 minutes, otherwise tissue damage could occur.

So to recap how to use this device:

1. Place the pump which can be run on batteries or pumped by hand over the penis.

2. Create a vacuum by pumping air out of the cylinder. The effect of the vacuum draws blood into the shaft of the penis which causes it to swell and become erect.

3. Next, with the aid of a suitable lubricant, slide the band down to the lower end of the penis.

4. Remove the pump following release of the vacuum.

5. Intercourse can now take place with the band in place.

6. Remember not to leave the band on for longer than 30 minutes.

Studies show that approximately 50 percent to 80 percent of men are more than satisfied with this type of device.

Who should use one of these devices?

These devices are considered safe and can be used by the following:

- Anyone suffering from a lack of blood flow to the penis.
- Anyone who has diabetes
- Anyone who has had surgery for colon or prostate cancer
- Anyone who suffers from depression or anxiety.
- These types of devices should not be used by the following:
- Anyone who is prone to a condition called priapism—a prolonged or painful erection that can last for several hours.
- Anyone who may have a significant congenital bleeding disorder.
- Anyone who has sickle cell anemia
- Different forms of leukemia
- Any other blood conditions.

Penile Prostheses

There are different types of penile prosthesis, but they all have the same goal—to enable you to achieve an erection so that you can have satisfactory intercourse. One important point! Neither the operation to insert the device or the device itself will compromise sensation, orgasm, ejaculation or the ability to urinate.

The penis contains two erection chambers. Whatever device is decided upon, paired cylinders will be inserted in these chambers. A less complicated form of penile prosthesis contains paired cylinders that are flexible. They are in fact made of medical grade silicone. They are semi rigid, and the idea is to bend the cylinders down to urinate and bend them upwards to have intercourse—simple!

Another type of penile prosthesis—which probably is the more natural feeling of the devices as it enables the individual to control size and rigidity—involves an inflatable penile prosthesis which is fluid filled and is inflated for an erection.

These inflatable devices are inserted into the erection chambers of the penis. Tubing connects these cylinders to a pump that is inserted inside the scrotum—the sac that contains the testicles.

This pump transfers a small amount of fluid into the cylinders for an erection. The fluid is transferred out of the cylinders when the erection is not needed anymore. This type of device is frequently referred to as a two part penile prosthesis. The first part is the paired cylinders and the second part is the pump.

There is also a three part inflatable penile prosthesis which consists of paired cylinders, a pump and an abdominal fluid reservoir. With the three pump device a larger volume of fluid is pumped into the paired cylinders when an erection is required, which is then pumped out when the erection is no longer needed.

How are penile prosthesis inserted?

Usually under anesthetic. A small cut is made either above the penis where it joins the abdomen or below the penis where it joins the scrotum. No tissue is removed and there is virtually no blood loss. Possibly one nights stay in hospital will be required.

The majority of men will experience a degree of pain for several weeks after the penile prosthetic insertion. This can however be minimized by reducing any form of exercise and taking a pain medication if required.

Usually after a period of four weeks, instruction can be given on how to use the device!

Are there any complications after surgery?

Approximately 1 to 3 percent of men will experience an infection. This is a big deal as it usually involves removal of the device.

Inflatable penile prosthetics can leak fluid into the body in about 10 to 15 percent of cases during the first five years. The fluid will not do any harm as it is a normal saline solution, which the body readily absorbs.

Where failure occurs, further surgery will be need to either repair the device or replace it.

I hope this chapter has answered some of your questions, and all that remains now if you feel that one of these devices is for you, is to go and see your doctor.

13. Naturopathy

When deciding how to deal with erectile dysfunction, many men often consider going down a more natural route, and naturopathy will come to mind. So what is naturopathy and how can it benefit someone with erectile dysfunction?

Naturopathic medicine—or to give it its more common name naturopathy is a specific system of primary health care that underscores prevention and the body's self-healing ability using natural therapies. A Naturopathic doctor (ND) will combine centuries-old knowledge and thinking that nature is the prime healer combined with present research on health issues and human body systems.

A Naturopathic doctor (ND) will focus his or her diagnosis on identifying the principle causes of a particular condition. Many naturopathic therapies are reinforced by research obtained from peer-reviewed journals, from many different disciplines, which includes naturopathic medicine, conventional medicine, clinical nutrition, European complementary medicine, homeopathy, pharmacognosy, phytotherapy, psychology and spirituality.

Therefore a naturopathic doctor will focus on the whole body by assessing emotional, mental, physical, genetics, environmental and social factors. As total health also includes spiritual health, a patient will be urged to follow their own spiritual path.

Disease prevention is a big part of naturopathy and your ND will discuss with you any genetic or hereditary conditions that you may be susceptible to, and if you are, he or she will suggest appropriate interventions to help prevent any possible illness.

A "wellness program" could be suggested to you. These programs are designed to maintain optimum health. Every person has a built-in wellness program—sometimes we just do not recognize it. Its core principle is having a belief in positive emotions, thoughts and positive actions. If a person can recognize these core principles, then there is every possibility that the body will more easily heal the disease than using direct medical intervention alone.

I am a great believer in using a natural approach where possible, so you might like to consult a qualified ND to discuss your erectile

dysfunction problem. An ND will certainly give you a sound medical examination, and will in all probability make some positive suggestions and treatment options for you to consider.

14. Treating Erectile Dysfunction
The Natural Way

In addition to medications and medical devices, there is a natural way that can be considered as well. The natural way can include: diet, exercise, vitamin and mineral supplements, and herbs.

Let us look at diet first. Your diet supplies the "fuel" in the form of various nutrients that your body needs to perform its billions of functions. Without adequate nutrition, dietary nutritional shortfalls can occur, which can have a profound effect on how you sleep, perform your daily tasks, and yes, your sexual activity as well.

There are various foods types to avoid if you want to enjoy good health and a healthy sex life. Foods to avoid—or eat in moderation include: junk food of all types which often contain excessive amounts of saturated fat as well as sugar, sodium and various additives. Also, avoid processed foods including meats that look so tempting at the deli counter, as well as all those dressings that tend to be put in or on just about everything. They may help the food taste good, but remember all this "good taste" will add to your waistline. Eat pizza in moderation—it is high in fat content; avoid desserts, including ice cream where possible.

So what should you eat? Start with increasing your intake of fresh fruits and vegetables. Not only are these good sources of fiber, but many of them are rich in vitamins, minerals, enzymes and fiber— something that is lacking in the "Western" diet. Also include "oily" fish twice each week if possible. Oily fish such as salmon, tuna, mackerel and sardines are rich in the essential fatty acid omega-3 EPA. If you don't fancy eating fish, then you could try a flax seed supplement which is from the flax plant. This is rich in omega 3, omega 6 and omega 9 essential fatty acids.

White meat is preferable to red meat, as red meat contains more fat. Remember if you are eating white meat to choose organic if possible, as many types of poultry contain growth promoters and have been injected with hormones. Also remove the skin before eating it, as this is where all the fat is.

Adequate fiber and grains are an important component of your diet. This can consist of lentils, legumes, beans of various kinds as well as cereals. Where cereals are concerned, ignore the pretty picture on the box, and look at the ingredient list instead. Look for one that you will enjoy eating, but it must have a high fiber content, otherwise, you might as well eat the box, as in some cases that could be more nutritious than the contents.

Fats are important as part of your diet, but eat them sparingly. Use non-trans-fat spread on your toast instead of butter. Be mindful that the cherry pie that looks so tempting in the supermarket is high in fat, sugar and possibly sodium. Think before you buy something—is this item really good for me, or does it just taste good?

Moving on to exercise. Exercise is good for you—but whatever exercise program you choose, you must enjoy doing it, otherwise you will get bored with it, and quit. Just 30 minutes each day, five days each week can have a profound effect on your health—and especially your sexual health.

Try to incorporate pelvic exercises into your exercise routine. Research shows that regular pelvic exercises help reduce the risk of developing erectile dysfunction. And if you are already suffering from erectile dysfunction, then regular pelvic exercises are a must.

Exercise has a positive effect on all the body systems—but especially your circulation, your glandular system (which is linked to your sexual health) and your immune system which helps to protect you from all manner of ailments from the common cold to fighting tumors which can be cancer forming.

However, it is best to discuss your proposed exercise program with your doctor to make sure it will be suitable for you, especially if you have any pre-existing medical conditions.

It is a well-known fact that due to intensive farming techniques as well as harvesting methods, the way crops and food are stored, and the way many foods are cooked, that nutrition quality and content tends to suffer. Remember, many plants can synthesize various vitamins themselves, as can the body, but minerals have to come from the soil. The body does not manufacture any minerals itself.

Therefore, if you have a dietary shortfall in vitamins and minerals, then supplementation may be in order. A good natural (not synthetic) multivitamin and mineral supplement could prove beneficial.

Always remember to discuss with your doctor before changing your diet or before starting a supplement or herbal program, especially if you have a pre-existing medical condition and / or are taking any form of medication.

In fact medications that are prescribed for hypertension (high blood pressure) diabetes and mental health conditions can cause sexual malfunctioning, as can being overweight, if you smoke, (smoking reduces muscle activity with the result that the penis finds it difficult to retain blood flow—and therefore an erection.)

Also drinking excess alcohol which has depressive effects can have a negative effect of your sexual activity.

And finally, it is important to reduce any anxiety and / or stress in your life. These feeling have the effect of reducing desire and potency. Try introducing meditation or yoga into your daily routine. Both of these can have a positive effect on your stress or anxiety levels. Also, talk to your partner about your concerns to help alleviate any tensions or misunderstandings in your relationship.

Herbal Supplements

Herbal preparations have been used for centuries to treat a multitude of health conditions. The following is a list for your consideration. All have proved beneficial for anyone suffering from erectile dysfunction. I have included a brief description of each one. You don't have to take them all. You may want to discuss this list with your health care provider if they are supportive of natural products, alternatively, you could consult a naturopathic doctor (ND) for advice.

Maca—is a root plant from Peru and is also known as Peruvian Ginseng, although it is not a member of the ginseng family.

Historically it has been used to boost energy and stamina and as an aphrodisiac to help improve sexual performance.

L. Arginine—is an amino acid which occurs naturally in dairy products, meat, poultry, fish and nuts. It is also available as a supplement.

Similar to the drug Viagra in that it is thought to enhance the actions of nitric oxide which has the effect of relaxing muscles surrounding blood vessels which supply blood to the penis. As a consequence, blood vessels in the penis dilate and allow blood to flow which could help maintain an erection.

In fact, one study published in 1999 in the journal BJU International involved 50 men with erectile dysfunction. This group either took 5 grams of L. Arginine each day or a placebo. After six weeks those who had taken L. Arginine showed an improvement in their sexual performance compared to those who had been taking a placebo.

L. Arginine is usually taken on a daily basis for erectile dysfunction.

Horny Goat Weed—is used in Chinese medicine. Studies show that Horny Goad Weed may work by elevating nitric oxide levels, which has the effect of relaxing muscles surrounding blood vessels in the penis, which has the effect of letting more blood flow, thus helping maintain an erection.

There is some evidence to suggest that this herb may modulate levels of various hormones including cortisol, testosterone and thyroid hormone, thus bringing low levels back within the normal range.

Cordyceps—a mushroom from Asia, has been used for thousands of years by practitioners of traditional Chinese medicine. Originally used to support the immune system and counter fatigue, it has gained much praise as a performance enhancer and energy booster.

Capsaicin/Capsicum—Capsaicin is the active ingredient in chili peppers which gives you a "hot" rush when eaten. Capsicum stimulates the circulatory system, thus increasing blood flow, and will give you a "warm felling".

Damiana—a plant native to the southern United States and Mexico, damiana has proved very popular as an aphrodisiac. Studies show that it contains compounds that mimic progesterone.

Ginkgo Biloba—an antioxidant herb, ginkgo helps stimulate the circulatory system and increase blood flow to the extremities. It could increase arousal in men and women by increasing blood flow to the genitals.

Ashwaganda—a member of the nightshade family, has long been used as an aphrodisiac in India.

Yohimbe—derived from the bark of an African tree and is the base material used in several pharmaceutical drugs to treat erectile dysfunction. Yohimbe is available as a supplement and can be purchased on the Internet and from health food stores.

This is not an exhaustive list of herbal supplements, but it will give you some information on a few of them. You can now do a little research yourself to see if any of these would be suitable for you.

But remember my advice—seek input from your doctor or a naturopathic doctor (ND) before taking any herbal products, especially if you are taking any medications for existing medical conditions.

15. Get The Support You Need

When a man is suffering from erectile dysfunction, one of the biggest mistakes he can make is to keep the problem to himself. It certainly is not the type of situation you want to discuss with everyone, but having a support system in place is one of the key steps to ensure you don't suffer from emotional and psychological issues as a result of it. If you are in a serious relationship, then you need to discuss the problem with your partner.

If your partner wishes to continue the relationship, then they will be supportive in your quest to resolve the problem. However, if they are not supportive, then perhaps this is the wrong relationship for you. Having the confidence to share such a sensitive issue with your partner can mean that they can help you to relax when sexual activity is underway. Tension and anxiety about your ability to perform sexually is one of the sure fire ways to not perform adequately. There are also additional ways to perform intimate acts in your relationship so neither of you need to feel deprived.

It is beneficial to have at least one close friend or family member who you can confide in about your problem. They can give you support and encouragement, and listen to your concerns and fears. But do make sure that you can really trust this person to keep your situation confidential. This way you will have the reassurance that other people won't find out about your condition, unless you choose to tell them yourself.

It is also worthwhile considering making your doctor part of your support system. Being a doctor with many patients, chances are that they have advised many different men with their erectile dysfunction concerns. In addition, your doctor will have plenty of support information to share with you which will make you realize that you are not the only person with the problem. They will also advise and work with you to help resolve the situation. However, if you feel uncomfortable about discussing this with your own doctor, then consider arranging an appointment with a different doctor instead.

Arranging an appointment with a counselor or therapist can be a good way to enhance your support system. In fact your doctor may recommend you schedule an appointment with one of these individuals if your erectile dysfunction problem is emotionally or psychologically related.

Have a look on the internet for support groups. This is a great way to get information and advice as you can remain anonymous. There are many online support groups that are free to join. You can read online discussion boards as well to see how other men are coping with the problem, and you can also join in the discussions as well should you choose to do so.

Sharing your concerns through an online support group can be very therapeutic for you. As everyone in the support group has the same problem, you can each support each other. In time you may develop some great friendship as well. Although erectile dysfunction may be the initial thing that introduced you, overtime you may discover that you have other things in common as well.

The support is out there is you want it. But you have to take the first step yourself—someone else is not going to do it for you. The more support you have, the easier it will be for you to cope with it and find a solution that will get your sex life back on track. So the decision is yours—why not make it today, and lessen the impact that erectile dysfunction is having on your life.

About The Author

Brian B Jacques started in business at a young age, and over the ensuing years, he has developed several very successful businesses. But his main interest for the past 40 years has been in natural health research and publishing.

Brian has presented seminars worldwide on such diverse subjects as Health Related issues, Motivation and Personal Development. In addition he has written numerous books, newsletters and articles on these subjects.

His very popular series of Mini Health Books has circulated widely around the world, and many more titles are in preparation.

Brian is a highly motivated individual, so much so that in 1985 he received a UK Industrial Society award for his work in the Motivation and Personal Development fields.

Brian has the following mottos:

- If something does not work out for you, then don't give up, but keep trying, trying, trying until finally you succeed.
- Success or failure in any endeavor is in your own hands.

Brian and his wife divide their time between East Yorkshire, UK and Florida, USA.

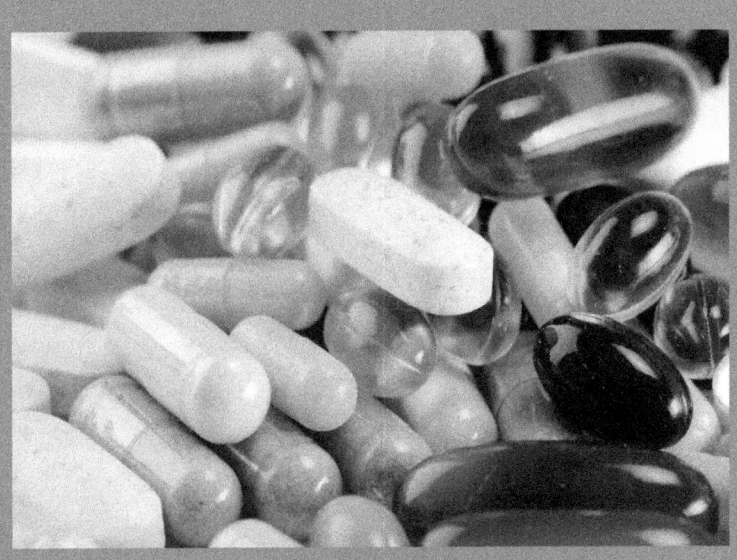

www.ingramcontent.com/pod-product-compliance
Lightning Source LLC
Chambersburg PA
CBHW071257280526
45788CB00004B/1740